Andrea Holst
Daniela Bolze

Colic

Causes, prevention and treatment

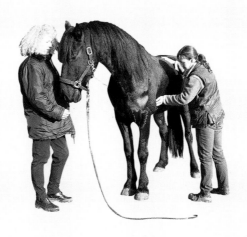

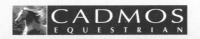
CADMOS
EQUESTRIAN

Contents:

Imprint

Copyright of original edition © 2003 by Cadmos Verlag
This edition © 2004 by Cadmos Equestrian
Translated by Ute Weyer MRCVS
Project management by Editmaster Co Ltd.
Design and composition: Ravenstein
Photographs: Daniela Holst
Printed by Grindeldruck

ISBN 3-86127-945-2

What is colic?

The word stems from the Greek word *colon,* meaning large intestine. Colic describes all types of abdominal pain. It is not a diagnosis, but just expresses the symptom "belly ache". Colic pain is usually felt in the gastro-intestinal tract.

The horse's digestion

Anatomy and facts

As we know, the horse is a herbivore. This means that it must digest cellulose, a particularly difficult and sensitive process.

When we talk about the digestive system of the horse, we include all the associated organs involved in the process, from eating to defecation, lips to anus. It is therefore a very complex affair.

The oral cavity consists of lips, mucus membranes, palate, tongue, and teeth. The adult horse has between 36 and 44 teeth. Then there are the salivary glands, the larynx, and the oesophagus down to the stomach. Compared to the horse's overall size, its stomach is relatively small, with a capacity of only 8–15 litres. Therefore, the horse needs to eat small but frequent amounts of food. Because of their anatomy, horses cannot vomit.

The small intestine is divided into three parts: duodenum, jejunum, and ileum. The duodenum is about one metre long, the jejunum about 25 metres and the ileum around 70 centimetres. It is up to 7 centimetres wide. Since the ileum has a very strong muscular wall, a blockage between ileum and caecum can develop. The caecum produces various gases that must not enter the small intestines, as they would harm the digestive procedures and extend the small intestines too much. The caecum is about one metre long, and can hold up to 33 litres. It is located in the right side of the abdomen. Caecal digestive noises can be easily heard from the right flank.

Caecum and colon work as "fermenting chambers" for the digestion of cellulose. All herbivores have to break down cellulose, which is difficult and prone to disturbances. The colon consists of three parts. The first part, the ascending colon, is three to four metres long with a diameter of 10 to 50 centimetres, with a capacity of up to 80 litres. The second part, the transverse colon, is short and narrow and presents an area prone to impactions. The third part, the descending colon, is two and a half to four metres long. In this part the droppings are already formed.

The final sections are the rectum with a length of 25 centimetres, and the anus.

All parts of the intestines – the measurements given are those of the average horse – are contained in the abdominal cavity in their own special locations and are held in place by a loose "net". Indeed, the intestines are held in place so loosely that rolling with distended guts can sometimes lead to lethal twists or displacements.

In addition to the actual intestinal tract there are also accessory glands, like the liver. The liver weighs about 5 kg and produces, in addition to enzymes etc., about 10 litres of bile per day. The bile is released into the intestines and is part of the fat digestion process. Unlike humans, horses have no gall bladder. The pancreas produces digestive enzymes, which are discharged into the small intestines.

What happens to food inside the horse?

If only one of these organs – and that includes the teeth – does not work properly, a colic with lethal consequences can develop.

The horse chews and breaks down its food roughly with its teeth and mixes it with saliva. The food is then transported through the oesophagus to the stomach. Here the food is digested further and then moved to the small

The gastro-intestinal tract

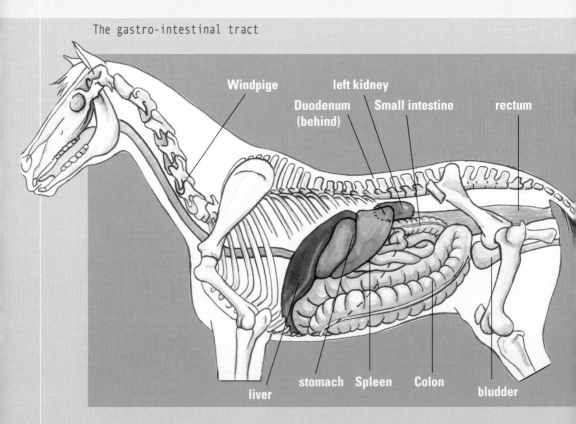

Windpige left kidney Duodenum (behind) Small intestine rectum

stomach Spleen Colon

liver bludder

intestines. The enzymes in the intestine break down the liquid pulp even more. The fermenting chambers of caecum and colon follow after the small intestines. The cellulose is broken down here in a complicated procedure. In the last part of the large colon, water is reabsorbed and the faeces are formed. During the passage through the gut, nutrients permeate through the intestinal wall into the blood stream. From the first lip and tongue contact down to the anus, the food is transported by muscle contractions through the body. In order to guarantee undisturbed digestion, the horse should be allowed to rest one to two hours after eating. The length of the resting period depends on the amount of food consumed.

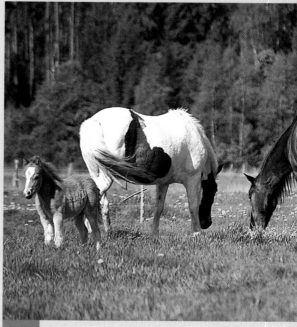

Left to their own devices, horses would eat gras 24 hours a day – not beneficial for the health of most breeds.

Natural habits of the horse

The horse's evolution as an animal of flight, living on the open steppes, is mentioned in most books about the keeping and training of horses, and it is a fact that cannot be sufficiently stressed. The actual conditions in some riding stables and studs, however, show that not everyone can be aware of this fact. The evolutionary development of the domesticated horse has only emphasised its nature as an animal of flight, and so it is important that their living and feeding conditions are appropriate.

The body of a flight animal is always poised to flee, run and move quickly at a second's notice – tendons, muscles, lungs, heart and digestion. This conflicts with having an overfull abdomen.

When left in their natural conditions, horses will eat small portions for up to 16 hours a day. While eating, they will walk slowly forward with their heads lowered. Horses have to tear out bunches of grass up to 50,000 times a day in order to satisfy their requirements. In the wild, they can walk for 10 kilometres just eating. The horse's digestive organs are designed to process fodder permanently in combination with continuous slow exercise. Horses rest in between meals, preferably close together in small groups. They sleep only for a maximum of 20 minutes stretched out on their sides, and only where and when they feel safe and secure.

Optimal feeding of domesticated horses

Be honest: who can feed their horses in an optimal way? In most stables horses are fed twice, at best three times, a day. The rest of the day they spend in their stables. Free exercise is allowed – if they are lucky – for a short time on a muddy paddock in the winter and often on their own. Many stables use shavings, so no straw is available and good hay is rare – instead they are fed lots of hard feed. These animals are a long way from continuous grazing and slow exercise – and as far from a healthy feeding regime. In the long term, incorrect stable management will lead to more or less obvious health problems.

Make sure, when selecting a yard, that your horse has access to fodder all day long. Depending on how chubby your horse is, this can be straw or hay/haylage. Fodder must be free of fungus, clean and without contamination or dirt. The food should be eaten from the floor and not from hayracks that are fitted high up on the wall. An open stable, where the horse can and has to walk between eating, resting and watering areas is most suitable. If that is not possible, the horse should be able to exercise freely for several hours a day in a sufficiently sized paddock, ideally with some

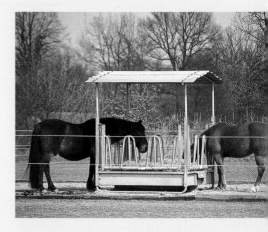

Optimal feeding: the horse has access to dry fodder all long without fighting and with sufficient exercise in between.

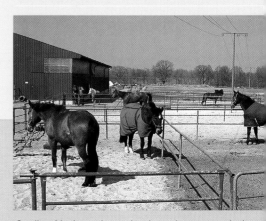

Small paddocks are better than boxes but are no substitute daily exercise.

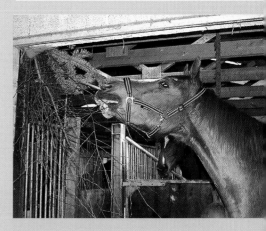

If a horse has to be stabled, edible foliage should be made available for chewing.

companions. Paddocks that are too small and muddy do not encourage horses to exercise, and they only stand around, as they would in a box. The only advantage is fresh air.

Split the hard feed into smaller portions, at least three, better even five. Also, check the actual demand for hard food, as many horses are fed far too much.

If your horse has to be bedded on shavings for health reasons, offer it branches and edible foliage to offset boredom and as a food "placebo", accompanied of course by sufficient amounts of fodder several times a day.

Care should be taken that horses have something to eat when loose in sandy paddocks, otherwise they tend to eat the sand. But do not let them eat from the muddy ground, because that way they will swallow sand anyway.

Make sure that your horse can eat without fear of the food being taken away again. This can be a problem not only in open stables but also in enclosed boxes, where neighbouring horses can threaten each other over food. You should try to either find a more placid neighbour, or feed your horse in the opposite corner so that direct contact can be avoided.

Tip

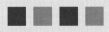

Feeding hard food in an open stable without separate boxes can be difficult. A cheap option allows a stress-free feeding time for all horses: remove the metal handles from an ordinary 10-litre bucket. Pierce a hole in their place and fit a length of rope through them. At feeding times, the rope is then placed behind the horse's ears, with the horse's mouth in the bucket. Even if a higher-ranking horse wants to chase away a lower-ranking one, the underdog flees with the feed "on board", and this type of jealousy will soon stop.

Remove the bucket promptly, as some horses will try to drink with it in place, thus causing the bucket to fill up with water and possibly cover the nostrils.

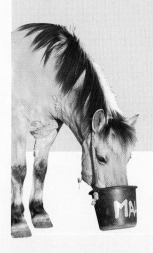

Causes of colic

There are many reasons why a horse may develop colic. The better these are known, the easier it is to treat and avoid them.

Stress

Horses react much more to external factors than riders and owners realise. They can feel joy, sorrow and – especially – stress, in the same way we can. If the relationship between horse and human is particularly close, the animal will even react directly to a person's mood. Reactions are also comparable: from tense muscles, mood swings (dislike, nervousness, and sorrow), to colic.

Triggers of stress can be:
- new stable or field
- fights over food
- loss of companion/owner
- performance-related (stress during competitions, very demanding work)
- hectic and loud environment
- stressed rider/owner
- generally nervous horses
- too much or too little going on in the stable (personal preference)
- dislike of stable mates.

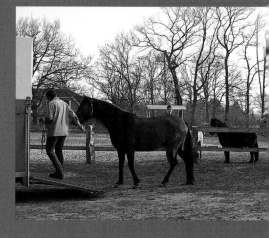

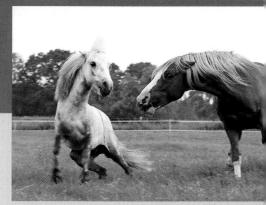

Continuous ranking fights can be stressful enough to cause colic in some horses. (Photo: Kristina Wedekind)

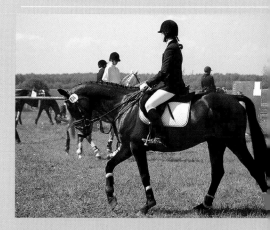

Not all horses cope well in a competition environment. Some become very nervous – colic risk!

Lack of exercise

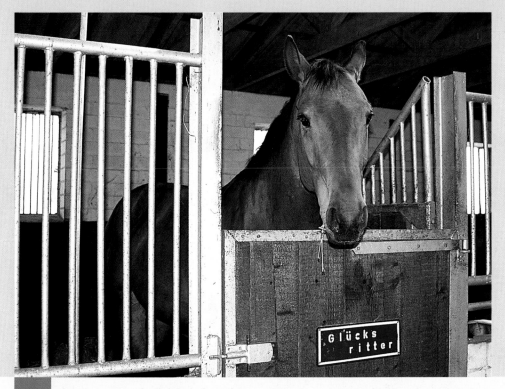

A common cause of colic is lack of exercise, which no horse should ever suffer from.

As mentioned before, the horse is a flight animal. Its whole organism is designed to move continuously and to be able to flee at any moment. Therefore, the horse requires exercise in order to feel well; this varies according to breed and age. Only then can all organs function properly – this includes the digestive system. When talking about exercise we mean DAILY exercise, and not twice a week when it fits in with the owner's other commitments. This is especially important for stabled horses. Open stable management allows the horse to decide for itself how much exercise it wants, but only when the paddock is large enough with suitable ground. Optimal and healthy digestion requires exercise – this applies to humans as well, as many people know from their own experience.

If it is not possible to provide your horse with regular and sufficient exercise, it is important to increase the work gradually and not gallop around the countryside or ask for high performance in the school or jumping arena without an adequate warm-up phase (at least 15 minutes at a relaxed walk).

Endoparasites

More than half of all colics are partly or even entirely due to endoparasites. These include tapeworms, ascarids and bots. First, endoparasites compete with the horse for nutrients. Severely infected horses remain thin, despite an adequate food supply, and their abdomen is distended ("worm belly"). Horses become emaciated and show signs of nutrient deficiencies. Secondly, endoparasites migrate through the horse's body. It is not only the gastro-intestinal tract that is damaged, but other organs too (e.g. liver and lungs). The greater the worm burden, the more problems they can cause; horses can die from worm infestation. A colic caused by endoparasites can be fatal.

It is most important to worm a horse at least four times a year in order to keep parasites to a minimum. Obviously, the more endoparasites inside the horse, the more will be damaged or killed by the wormer. These damaged or dead endoparasites can present two big problems: first, the development of toxins in the gastro-intestinal tract; secondly, the worms can form conglomerates, which are pushed with difficulty through the partly narrowed gut. Therefore, regular and frequent worming is kinder to the horse. Colics that develop after administering a wormer are not a reaction to the actual drug, but to the amount of dying or damaged endoparasites inside.

Not only do horses need to be wormed at least four times a year, but different wormers should also be used, to avoid the development of resistance. There are four phar-maceutical groups of wormers: avermectine, pyrimidine, benzimidazole based groups and praziquantel. Care must be taken to select a wormer from a different pharmaceutical group and not just change to a different proprietary brand containing the same active ingredient. Let your vet advise you. In the winter (December/January), it is important to choose a wormer that will kill bots. Thorough stable and pasture management is vital in order to minimise endoparasite infection, but hygiene is no substitute for regular worming.

The contents of a wormer are more important than the trade name and they should be changed regularly, to guarantee the effectiveness.

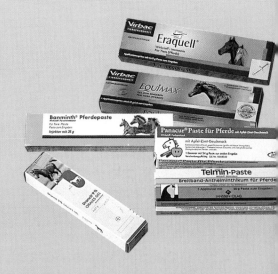

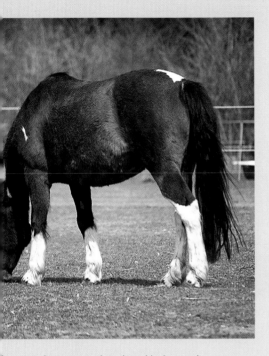

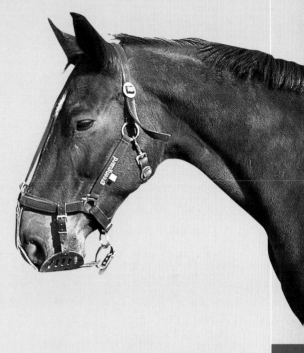

Overgrazed pastures and sandy paddocks greatly increase the risk of sand colic.

Horses that will not stop licking soil should wear a muzzle when outside – still a better option than being stabled.

Sand

Ingestion of sand is a repeated cause of colic. A horse can swallow too much sand and soil when kept on an overgrazed pasture, where it will pull out and eat the grass roots with the soil. Horses are especially at risk in the spring when grazing on pasture with patchy growth. Feeding hay from the ground also encourages the ingestion of sand. If there is insufficient food available, horses eat sand in an attempt to reach the last remaining piece of grass. There are also some horses which eat sand deliberately. In these cases, alternative chewing materials should be offered (straw, twigs) or a muzzle fitted, as long as mineral or trace element deficiency can be ruled out as the cause of this behaviour.

A word of caution:
Sometimes, good intentions can cause colic. Horses in rain-soaked paddocks pull twigs through the mud and thus eat a lot of sand stuck on the bark, which can lead to a sand colic. Here it is recommended that the twigs be tied to the fence, trough or wall.

Stabled horses can also eat too much sand if food or bedding material is contaminated with it. It is therefore very important to store the feed in a clean area.

A regular treatment with so-called flea seed can be used as prevention. The seeds swell in the gastro-intestinal tract and wash out sand from the intestines. Sand is then passed out together with the seeds.

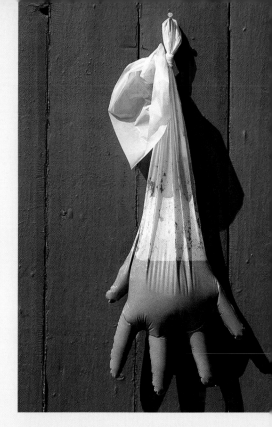

With a simple sediment test you can find out if your horse is eating too much sand.

Tip

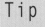

If your horse seems at risk of eating sand, you should test the faeces regularly for sand. Ask your vet for some long examination gloves, or take a plastic bag (e.g. small bin liners, hung up with one corner pointing down). Collect some droppings and fill the glove with water up to the wrist area. Make sure the droppings were not collected from sandy ground. Mix the contents well and let the glove hang, fingers pointing down, undisturbed overnight. You can then feel for sand particles at the bottom of the glove (or in the corner of the bag). This is called a sediment test.

Feeding problems

Most painful colics are caused by what and how you feed your horse.

Quality of food
Hard food:
Whether you feed grain, nuts, mix or similar, horse feed must be clean and free of fungus, mites, bacteria and dirt. Check the sell-by date. In order to guarantee your feed remains in good condition until this date, it should be stored in dry, mould free containers, which are also secure against mice and horses. Open food bags are an invitation to rodents.

Fodder:

Silage, haylage, hay or straw also have to be free of mould and dirt. Hay should be stored for at least two, or preferably even four months, before it is fed to horses. The fermenting process, which takes place during drying, has to be completed first. The older the hay, the more nutrients it loses, which must be taken into account when calculating the required amounts. On the other hand, this can be of advantage when feeding "good doers", or horses that are prone to laminitis.

Make sure when buying or making haylage/silage that it is well wrapped and that the bales are undamaged. They should be placed on their flat side immediately afterwards to minimise the risk of fungal growth. Opened haylage or silage bales should be used within a maximum of two weeks, depending on humidity and weather conditions.

Quantity

The amount of food that is required depends upon the individual horse; on its condition, required performance, breed, metabolism and the nutritional content of the feed. The main part of the diet should consist of fodder. Far less high-energy food is required than is generally believed. The majority of riding club horses and hacks that are being ridden for one hour a day in walk could live on just fodder, minerals and salts, without an ounce of hard feed. Therefore, the amount of hard feed (nuts, grain, mix) should be kept to a minimum. The horse's wild ancestors did not have access to this type of food and its gastrointestinal tract is not ideally equipped to digest it. (A high intake of energy food with only small amounts of fodder increases the risk of gastritis and stomach ulcers.) A 500 kg horse will need about one bale of hay per day (about 9–15 kg, depending on its quality). If your horse is a "good doer" and tends to become chubby, the energy content of the fodder should be low: straw, last year's hay, this year's hay, haylage. The bulk volume should not be decreased, as the intestines need to be kept active.

Feeding management

It is very important for a horse to have food available almost continuously, but this is difficult to achieve for various reasons – lack of personnel, or because the horse will simply become too fat. Horses should, however, be fed at least twice a day, otherwise someone else should take over the feeding regime for the health of the animal. If hard feed is given, this should be done about 30 minutes after the horse has had some fodder. The intestines can then break down concentrated hard feed more efficiently and will cope with the often heated or chemically treated food more easily. If you have to change feed, whether it is the type of hard feed, brand or fodder, it should be done gradually and never from one day to the next. Try to extend the change over period for up to a week, by increasing the proportion of "new" food until it replaces the old one.

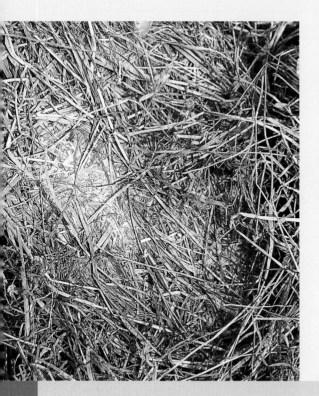

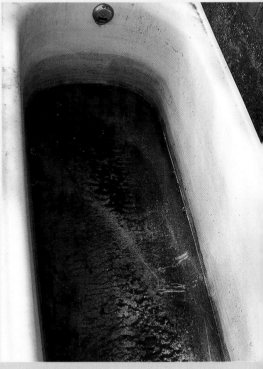

Rotten fodder should never be part of the horse's menu…

… nor dirty drinking water. Both can cause colic.

Water

Water for horses must be of drinking water standard, and the quality should be analysed if the water stems from natural sources or wells. Often E. coli bacteria etc. can be found that are as damaging for horses as for humans. Water must not be contaminated by algae, animal faeces or dirt. It is very important that horses have access to water at ALL times throughout the year, especially on hot summer days, and very cold days. This is particularly important for lactating mares.

Infections

Infections of the gastro-intestinal tract can cause colic. For example, Salmonella can be transmitted via contaminated feed and from horse to horse.

In many cases, other infections like respiratory or generalised infections can trigger a colic attack. In this situation horses often lose their appetite due to fever or coughing and they eat intermittently. The gut is not sufficiently supported and colic can develop. It is without problems. Sometimes the growing foal pushes certain parts of the intestines to the edge of the abdominal cavity where there is not enough space – colic develops.

It is important to allow pregnant mares to eat small, frequent and easily digestible meals.

It is rare but should be mentioned – sometimes labour can induce colic because of the increased pressure in the abdomen.

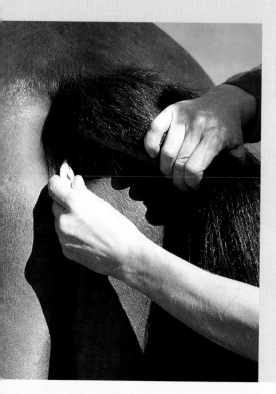

A raised body temperature is a sign of infection.

The growing foal in its mother's abdomen can cause bellyache as well as induce labour. "Birth" colic can develop.

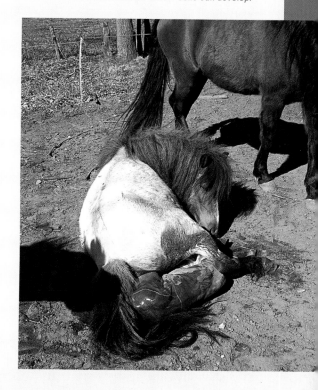

vital to check your sick horse for any signs of colic, and to pay particular attention to its nutrition.

Pregnancy and birth

No pregnant woman needs an explanation as to why mares in foal are prone to colics: there is simply not much space left in the abdomen. The gut has less room, and food cannot be transported through the lumen

Hormonal changes

Some mares suffer from colic every time they are in season – very much to the despair of their owner. These colics are partly due to hormonal changes but can also be caused by abnormalities of the ovaries (e.g. tumours).

Abdominal growth

An abdominal growth can be caused by an abscess, tumour or bruise. They limit the free movement of intestinal sections, which can lead to colic. It is therefore important to let the attending vet know if your horse has been involved in a fight.

Adhesions

Certain organs (e.g. the liver and the pancreas) can stick to each other. This can be caused by congenital anomalies, inflammations or surgical processes. In these cases the intestines cannot move and work freely.

Hernias

Hernias can be situated in the groin or navel area. They can also occur along the whole abdominal midline. Usually they are congenital, but hernias can also develop after abdominal surgery or trauma. Gut loops trapped in these hernias can result in severe colics. The blood supply to these incarcerated loops is interrupted and they die off, which can be fatal.

Foreign bodies in the gastro-intestinal tract

Although rare when sufficient food is available, horses have been known to eat stones, plastic or other foreign bodies. These cannot be broken down, and block the intestines. Some can produce toxins under the influence of digestive enzymes.

Foreign bodies can also develop from inside when salt and crystals contained in the food bind together and grow into stones. These prevent food from passing through the lumen.

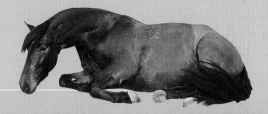

Chronic inflammation

Chronic inflammation of the gut can be caused by bacteria (e.g. Salmonella), viruses or sand. Sand acts like sandpaper and destroys the villi on the intestinal surface.

Crib-biting

Crib-biting is an expression of psychological stress, and results in too much air in the gastro-intestinal tract. Normal gut function is disturbed and horses tend to develop colic. It is vital that these horses are offered sufficient amounts of fodder.

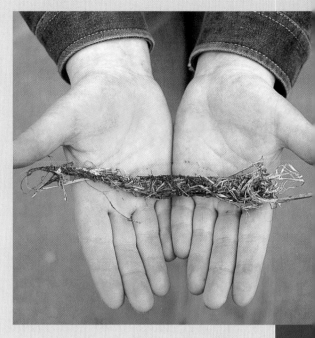

A masticated lump of hay is a definite sign of teeth problems. A vet needs to examine the teeth and treat them as necessary.

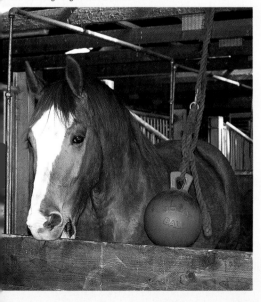

Crib-biters like this one are at risk of suffering from colic due to swallowing large amounts of air.

Dental abnormalities

Teeth are the start of the digestive system. If food is not sufficiently chewed and prepared, indigestion will follow. Sharp hooks, missing teeth, caries, inflammation of the gums or teeth roots, all impede adequate chewing of the food. Watch your horse every now and then when it is eating. Does it eat all the hard feed? Do food particles drop out of its mouth? Does it form masticated lumps of food (depending on their size, small cigar-shaped rolls)? Every horse, whether it is a riding horse or elderly and inactive, should have its teeth examined annually by a vet. If necessary the teeth

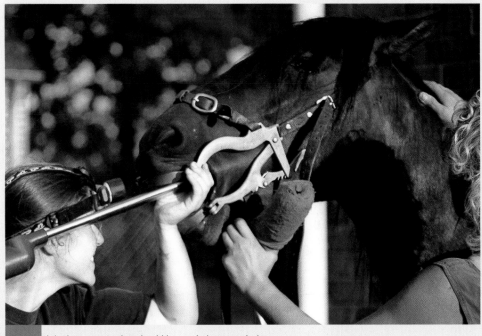

*It looks gruesome but should be carried out regularly –
teeth rasps.*

must be treated. In the wild, horses can
starve to death if their teeth are no longer
healthy – which unfortunately still happens
in stables, despite the horses having access
to plenty of food.

Weather influences

Veterinarians can expect to cancel their
evening engagements during certain weather conditions. Many horses go down with
colic when the weather changes significantly. If these conditions prevail, owners
should prepare themselves: sufficient exer-

cise, careful feeding, and rugs, depending
on temperatures.

Poisonous plants

It is possible that wild horses are able to dis-
tinguish between "good" and "bad" food. Our
domesticated horses, however, especially
those living on a restricted diet, are no longer
capable of doing so. They wolf down anything
they can get – sometimes even plants that
are poisonous and can cause colic. Make
sure that no such plants grow around the stable, in your field or along the fences; also

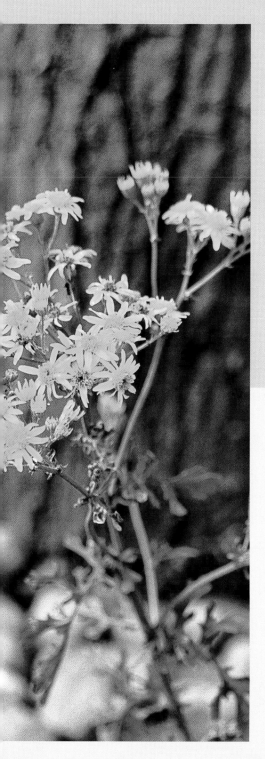

agwort

check the type of twigs offered for chewing, and shredded wood used in the riding arena. When hacking out, be careful what your horse may try to eat along the way.

If your horse swallows one of the following plants (the list is not comprehensive, but limited to colic-related plants) let your vet know, so he/she can administer an antidote if necessary and be prepared for the type of colic which may develop. Call the vet out immediately. Move your horse away from the source of poison. Do not give any hard feed, just fodder if anything at all. The vet can empty the stomach and increase passage through the intestines by giving salts and oils. Charcoal will bind the toxins.

Colic-inducing poisonous plants:

Black locust:
Planted in many gardens. Induces spasmodic colic.

Ragwort:
Grows in fields. Can cause impaction.

Autumn crocus:
Causes colic with severe bloody diarrhoea.

White cedar, box, laburnum:
Popular bushes. They all cause spasmodic colic.

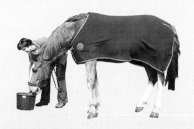

Colic symptoms

No matter what type of colic we are dealing with, there are certain common symptoms, and horses vary in how they react to pain. It can be breed-related – highly bred horses are often more sensitive. Not all symptoms are present at the same time. The next chapter will describe the various symptoms for every colic type.

   If you have the slightest suspicion of colic, call your vet immediately. An episode of colic can pass without veterinary intervention, but we know from experience that this is the exception and that an untreated colic can be fatal. The sooner a colic patient is treated, the better is the chance of recovery.

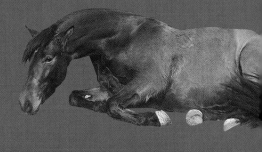

Horses that often lie down, get up, roll and appear to be in pain are very likely to be suffering from colic.

Symptoms

- Loss of or diminished appetite.
- Pawing the ground, box-walking, turning round in circles, lying down and getting up again.
- Rolling.
- Turning round to look at its abdomen.
- Kicking the abdomen as if there were flies.
- Swishing the tail as if trying to chase away insects.
- Flehming.
- A pained expression: the grooves above the eyes deepen. Nostrils are slightly pulled up, the muzzle is tense and pupils are dilated. Some horses even grind their teeth.
- Sweating. With some colics the sweat pours down the body.
- Most horses are restless but some are reluctant to move. They stand in one place, are dull and depressed.

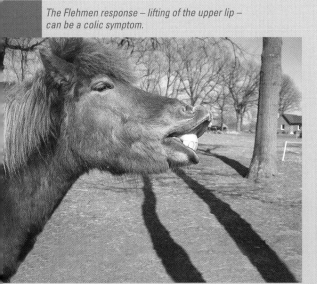

The Flehmen response – lifting of the upper lip – can be a colic symptom.

Types of colic

- Spasmodic colic
- Gas colic
- Impaction
- Displacement
- Arterial blockage
- Internal obstructions

The causes and symptoms listed below describe the most common signs of a particular type of colic. This does not mean that other symptoms cannot be displayed as well.

Spasmodic colic

Causes: feeding problems (low-quality food, changes in food) or weather influences.

Symptoms: initially gut sounds will increase, frequent faeces, often diarrhoea. The horse is restless, lies down, gets up again, rolls. Gut sounds and production of faeces cease during the course of the colic. The horse settles down. The vet can feel tense gut loops on a rectal examination.

Prognosis: favourable if treated early enough.

Gas colic

Causes: extensive gas production in the gastro-intestinal tract. The lumen of the affected section distends significantly, caus-

ing pain. The gas rises, often leading to a displacement of the gut. Gas production can be so severe that the extended intestines press against the diaphragm, making breathing difficult. Intestinal veins can be compressed, compromising the blood supply. This can cause the gut to die.

This process is triggered by:
- Fermenting feed types, e.g. clover, freshly cut grass, lawn mower cuttings, withered hot greens, potatoes, very fresh hay and many more.
- Obstructed intestines. Normal gas will build up, as it can no longer escape.

Symptoms: these colics usually develop shortly (within an hour) after eating or following a colic with intestinal obstruction. Horses show various stages of discomfort. The abdomen can extend on one or both sides (especially in the flanks). Initially, some gas is still being emitted. The animal produces plenty of droppings and there are distinct gut sounds, as the gas acts as an amplifier. The production of faeces will later stop and gut sounds reduce until they disappear.

If gases are trapped in the stomach it is possible that the horse will occasionally burp. Breathing is laboured, the horse sweats, and the pulse rate is elevated. On a rectal examination, the gas-filled loops can be clearly felt. Some parts of the intestines can be so full of gas that the original obstruction can no longer be felt.

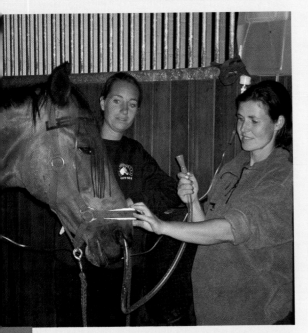

A stomach tube can help release trapped gas from the stomach. In this case, the tube was left in place for two days and the horse was saved without surgical intervention. (Photo Maren Schlack)

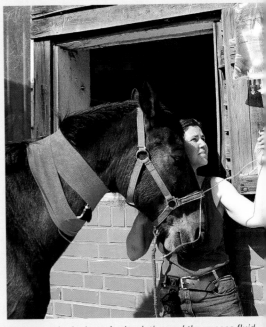

Drips sustain the horse's circulation and the excess fluid also supports gut function and can soften up dry intestinal contents.

Prognosis: must be very guarded. If gas production is rapid and extensive, this type of colic can be fatal within a few hours.

Impaction

This is the second most common colic type after spasmodic. The intestinal contents thicken to form a mass which can no longer be transported through the gut without difficulty. This causes the intestines to expand. Colon and caecum are most commonly affected, whereas a small intestinal impaction is very rare.

Causes: too much and the wrong type of food (hard fibre hay, too much straw, bedding material, wood, soil or sand that horses eat out of boredom); insufficient chewing (greedy eating, fodder cut too short, grass nuts, pellets, lawn mower cuttings); dental problems; lack of exercise; slow gut movements – especially in older horses; abnormal gut flora; gut paralysis; obstructions; spasms – leading to a narrowing of the lumen.

Symptoms: in cases of the rare small intestine impaction, horses break out in a heavy sweat, but sweat only mildly when colon or caecum are affected. Symptoms are not very obvious and the horse may still eat, although probably less than usual. It may sound a paradox: especially when suffering from an impaction, horses can develop diarrhoea. The reason for this is that only water and very small particles can get past the impaction, while a bigger and more solid mass becomes stuck.

Prognosis: if treated in time, the prognosis for colon and caecum impaction is favourable, but very guarded for small intestinal impactions.

Displacements

There are very different types of intestinal displacement. For example, a twist of one section around its axis or with other intestines; a volvulus; an intussusception. These can develop in the small or large intestines. The intestines can no longer move freely and the blood supply is often interrupted, and the intestinal lumen is narrowed.

Causes:

- The main reason is a severely increased peristaltic (muscle contraction) during a colic.
- Mechanical influences due to rolling.
- Sand – a heavy section pulls the intestine down.
- Gases – the intestines tend to move upwards.

Symptoms: usually colic signs (pain!), circulation problems, sweating. Initially, the peristaltic is increased, but this will later stop. Heart and respiration rates are elevated and body temperature is raised. The horse breathes superficially and is dehydrated (as a test, you can lift some skin on the neck and then let it go again. If the skin fold does not disappear immediately, the horse is dehydrated.)

On a rectal examination, the vet can usually feel a displacement, a secondary build up of gas, little to no faeces, and mucus in the rectum.

Treatment: conservative treatment is not usually sufficient and the horse must be taken to a clinic as soon as possible, where colic surgery will be performed. In the clinic, the horse will be put on a drip and treated with painkillers, relaxing medications, and the stomach will be emptied before surgery is carried out. During the last few years, anaesthesia and surgical techniques have

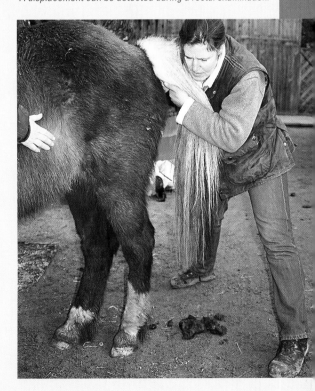

A displacement can be detected during a rectal examination.

improved considerably and success rates are increasing.

Prognosis: without surgical intervention a horse can die within twelve hours – or occasionally after a few weeks of illness. Horses operated on early have a good chance of recovery, but one has to remain cautious. The longer the displacement persists, the higher the risk of irreversible damage to the gut and the prognosis must be considered as guarded. A stable circulation greatly improves the chance of recovery.

Prophylaxis: the greater the delay in treating a colic, no matter how harmless it may appear, the greater the likelihood of a displacement following another type of colic. If the colic is treated properly within one to two hours of occurrence, the subsequent development of a displacement is rare.

Arterial blockage

Causes: Palisade worms, large strongyles. The larvae persist in the arterial walls and cause inflammation with a blood clot that narrows and later blocks the lumen of the artery. This thrombus can become detached from the wall and migrate as a so-called embolus into smaller arteries and cause blockages. The blood supply to the intestines is then disrupted and the gut fails to function properly.

Symptoms: this colic usually develops for no obvious reason, something as simple as a change of weather, feed etc. All colic

symptoms can be displayed and intestinal noises are usually present.

On a rectal examination the vet is unable to detect gas or abnormal intestines. Only in extremely severe cases does the gut fill with gas and tense up.

Treatment: in addition to normal colic treatment, the animal needs to be wormed with ivermectine-based wormers.

Prophylaxis: worming at least four times a year with a suitable wormer. Clean stable and pasture management.

Internal obstructions

Causes: intestinal stones, hard faeces, clumps of plant material, hairballs, haematomas, parasites.

Symptoms: the horse shows typical moderate colic symptoms over a long period (see "Colic symptoms"). Initially some droppings can still be produced, but this ceases during the course of the colic. On first examination the vet can feel a full colon and rectum, but latterly both will be empty.

Prognosis: without surgical correction the horse can deteriorate and die within one to two weeks.

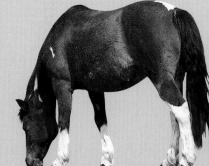

First aid until the vet arrives

Owners can do numerous things to help their horses until the vet arrives. In all cases, the vet needs to be called out.

This applies to all colic types:

- Take away all food immediately
- Depending on the time of year, put a thin rug on the horse, in order not to stress the circulation even more.
- Walk the horse gently (no lungeing or strenuous exercise).
- Contrary to popular opinion, do not let your horse roll. The gut can become twisted. This means that a formerly treatable colic now needs surgery – or may no longer be correctable.
- Calm your horse down and avoid any additional excitement and stress.

Horses suffering from colic should be walked gently without getting cold or tired.

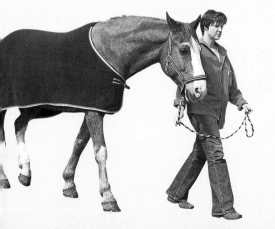

Colic examination

Each clinical examination must begin with a thorough history from the owner or groom. The vet has to learn as much as possible about the likely causes of the colic. The history should include information about feeding, droppings, sweating, exercise, and different or unusual occurrences. The owner can use the time until a vet arrives to gather these facts or, if necessary, to ask those who rode, fed or mucked out the horse.

The vet then examines the horse. He/she checks the size and shape of the abdomen and examines the abdominal cavity with a stethoscope. Sounds of the small and large intestines can be heard over the left flank, the caecum over the right flank. Noises should be audible in all areas during a two-minute period.

Abnormalities can be heard as reduced sounds, no sounds or sounds of less intensity. In some cases, however, increased frequency and intensity of sounds are indicative of a problem. The layman's ear pressed against the belly concluding "It gurgles, therefore it can't be colic" is simply wrong.

Auscultation of the heart – listening to it – provides another indication of the severity of the illness. A normal horse's heart beats between 36 and 40 times per minute; in colic patients this can be higher. When they reach 60 beats per minute, the situation can become life-threatening. The release of toxins from the gut can lead to heart murmurs.

The pulse should also be 36 to 40 beats per minute. This and colour of the mucus membranes are indicators of the patient's circulation. Normal mucus membranes are of a pale pink colour. Under abnormal circumstances they are often red, blue or "washed out".

A normal respiration rate is around 16 breaths per minute. During a colic, breathing is often laboured or increased and more costal due to the pain. The normal breathing type in horses (and humans) is costo-abdominal.

In addition to the body temperature (it should be between 37 and 38 degrees celsius), surface temperature is also of importance. During colic it can be normal, or show a hot or cold sweat. Horses in severe pain sometimes stand with cold sweat dripping off their whole body, often a sign of a small intestinal displacement.

Fresh droppings, if present, are examined thoroughly. The consistency and colour can give many clues. Some faeces are almost always in the rectum, which the vet can and must remove before a rectal examination. Only a vet should carry out this type of examination, as improper manipulation can lead to serious injuries. Very small horses and foals cannot be examined rectally due to their anatomical limitations.

Although only about 40% of the abdominal cavity can be explored manually, this can yield a lot of information. In a normal situation the vet can feel the spleen, part of the left kidney and the reno-splenic ligament in the left upper quarter; in mares also the left ovary and the left half of the uterus. In the right upper quarter the caecum can be felt, as well as the right ovary and right half of the uterus. In the lower parts the vet can find sections of the colon and the bladder; in stallions and geldings the inguinal canal.

During colic the veterinarian can detect extended loops of small intestines, gas-filled parts of caecum or colon, impacted sections, displacements or empty areas, swelling and/or displacement of the spleen, abscesses and tumours, rough surface of the peritoneum, muscular anomalies (too tense, too soft), injuries of the rectum, a severely filled bladder that cannot be emptied, or watery gut content.

A stomach tube is used for diagnostic and therapeutic purposes. As most horses will vehemently resist this procedure, sedation or the use of a twitch are advised.

A specially designed tube, approximately 120 centimetres long and up to 2 centimetres in diameter, is inserted through the nostril and the lower nasal passage to the larynx. This usually results in a swallowing reflex as the tube enters the oesophagus and then the stomach.

Diagnostics: stomach gases escape through the inserted tube and their smell and quantity will give the vet valuable clues. The stomach contents can be emptied (the stomach fluid is sucked out) and checked.

Treatment: emptying the stomach will release the pressure on the upper part of the small intestines. Unlike humans or dogs, horses are unable to vomit. Simply releasing the gases will relieve the stomach and therefore the pain. If the gases cannot escape either through the oesophagus or the small intestines, the stomach can, in extreme cases, burst.

The vet can examine a few blood parameters (thickness of the blood, leukocytes) at the stable yard. A more extensive blood test can reveal a great deal about the general condition of the horse or parasite infestation, and therefore possible causes of the colic.

Many colic patients need to be put on a drip that delivers saline solution, minerals and glucose intravenously. The amount dispensed can vary between 10 and 30 litres per day and this will stabilise the circulation and can loosen up impactions.

Preferably only performed in a clinic, a peritoneal tap can prove to be of significant diagnostic value. Fluid is extracted from the abdominal cavity by inserting a needle into the lower abdomen. The amount of fluid varies between three and 500 millilitres, depending on the type of illness of the horse. The quantity, but also the consistency, colour, smell, viscosity and content (blood cells, bacteria, food particles) can provide information as to the cause of colic. If a diagnosis remains unclear, even colic surgery can be used as a diagnostic means. This procedure is called an exploratory laparotomy. Sometimes the causes can be found immediately (gut loops, tumours etc) and can be corrected. If this is not possible,

the animal should be put down, as there is no chance of recovery.

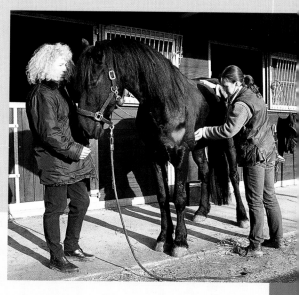

An absolute necessity during a colic examination is auscultation of heart and intestines, the rectal examination ...

... and a check of the mucus membranes as an indication of the circulation.

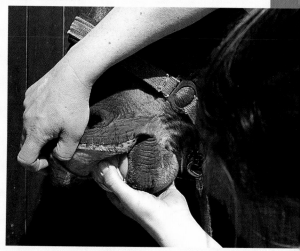

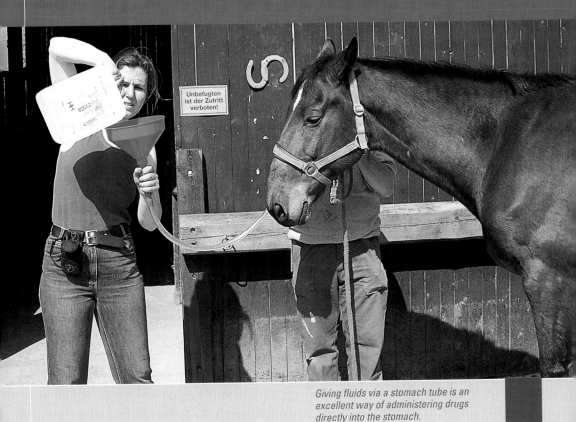

Giving fluids via a stomach tube is an excellent way of administering drugs directly into the stomach.

Treatment

What can the vet do in the stable?

After a thorough examination, the vet is limited to a few, albeit effective, therapeutic methods. Depending on the type of colic, the patient will receive spasmolytic drugs and painkillers.

The vet can administer medication (up to five litres of liquid paraffin, water, saline solution, charcoal) via a stomach tube directly into the stomach. The vet can also flush out the stomach. Colic patients need to be checked every two to four hours, as the effect of the injected drugs will wear off, and the horse must be monitored for persistent or recurrent colic symptoms.

What the owner has to do

After the vet has left the yard, the real work starts for the owner – this can be prolonged, and usually continues throughout the night.

The vet's instructions must be followed meticulously.

The following usually applies:

- It is very important that the horse does not eat any more food – not even straw. Therefore, every yard should possess some bales of shavings for emergencies, which can be used as bedding for colic patients for a few days. Many owners mean well and feed "only a handful", but even this is too much and can cause more harm than good. If shavings are not available and the horse is likely to eat its bedding, a muzzle should be used. The muzzle has to fit well and must not be too loose; otherwise the horse can get caught up in it. This is best combined with a well fitting head collar.

- The horse should – as long as the circulation allows this – be walked gently to encourage gut motility.

- It is very important to check your horse thoroughly about two to four hours after the administration of painkillers, to see if colic symptoms persist or recur. In this case, the vet needs to be called out again.

- Food must be introduced again very slowly. Small amounts of hay should be given no sooner than 24 hours after the colic and then increased over the course of a week to the normal amount. Hard food should be introduced in small amounts 48 hours later. After an impaction, it is especially important that the horse is fed small amounts of fodder to allow it to restore its normal gut function.

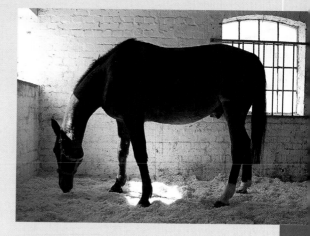

The horse should be stopped from eating at the first sign of colic. Either by keeping it in a stable on shavings ...

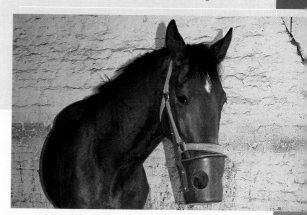

... or, if that is not possible, by using a muzzle which makes eating impossible.

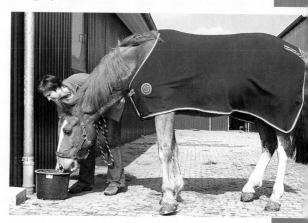

The horse should be offered water, preferably from a bucket and not from automatic drinkers.

- The animal should be allowed to exercise slowly, preferably in a sandy paddock. Do not turn it out in an over-grazed field where it can still eat the odd bit of grass. The horse should not be subjected to any strenuous work immediately after colic.
- Keep your horse out of any draught. If necessary put a rug on (on cold days, in cold wind).

Make sure your horse has access to plenty of clean water.

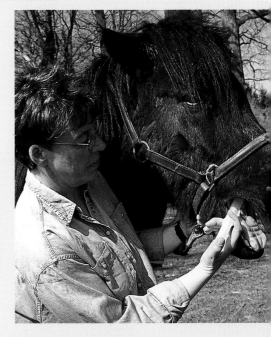

Homoeopathic drugs are dissolved in water and squirted into the mouth at regular intervals.

Tip

After a colic, it is beneficial to offer the horse freshly mixed mash in order to make feeding and digestion easier, but make sure the mash is soaked long enough before feeding it.

Alternative methods of support

Nux vomica C30 (globuli)

When spotting the very first colic signs, homoeopathic treatment may in certain cases ease the symptoms. It does not substitute a vet's visit! Call the vet before you start the nux vomica treatment, because even 60 minutes can be life-saving when dealing with colic.

Dissolve 3 - 5 globuli of nux vomica C30 in a glass of water. Use only a non-metallic tool to stir, as any metal will interfere with the medication. Pull up 15–20 millilitres of water in a syringe and squirt it into the horse's mouth. If you do not have a glass handy in which to dissolve the globuli you can place the globuli directly between lip and gums. Repeat this three times every 20 minutes.

Nux vomica-Homacord (liquid preparation)

A homoeopathic combination with a broader spectrum than pure nux vomica. Administer 20 drops in case of a suspected colic, 30 drops in an acute onset. The effect has to be immediate!

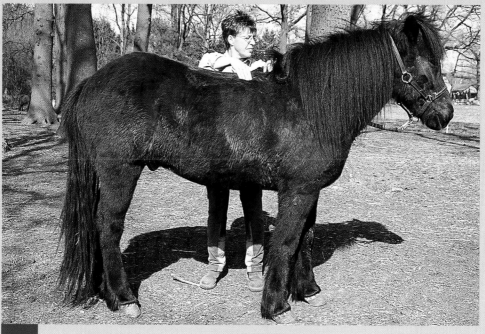

Instinctively you may want to ease your horse's pain by massaging the belly, but it is better to divert the energies along the back and stroke them out.

Massage:
You can ease your horse's pain by activating the meridians to the left and right of the spine. Do not massage the abdomen directly, as it will only concentrate the energy. Instead, massage with gentle pressure from your index fingers the area from the neck down to the tail on either side of the spine. Work evenly .

Colic surgery

Colics that cannot be treated by the above mentioned methods need surgical intervention. Among these are severe impactions, displacements and twists, sand colics and sometimes spasmodic colics.

During surgery the horse is placed on its back under general anaesthesia and the abdomen is opened via a midline incision. If the gut is displaced or twisted, its position may then be corrected. Should sections have died off, they will have to be resected; the chances of recovery will be poor.

Impacted or blocked intestines will be massaged in order to try and shift the gut content. If that does not help, the gut must be opened up, which is often the case when dealing with sand colics. In some cases surgeons have emptied out a whole wheelbarrow-full of gut contents. Adhesions are separated, tumours or abscesses removed.

In the case of spasmodic colic, the gut can be vented by inserting a trochar on a standing, sedated horse, without having to open the abdomen.

Colic surgery requires a lot of personnel and not all clinics are able to perform them. Find out where your nearest suitably equipped clinic is located and have directions and telephone numbers in your, hopefully well-equipped, first aid box.

Prognosis/risk patients

Even a harmless-looking colic can be fatal, as it is a very dynamic process. It is therefore crucial to involve the vet straight away.

A spasmodic colic, if treated early on, has a better prognosis than an impaction.

The majority of displacements cannot be corrected without surgery (but there are always exceptions). Surgery without opening up the intestines usually has a favourable prognosis. Problems start when parts of the gut have to be resected or opened.

Prophylaxis

Colic should always be considered as a warning sign to the owner. It should be used as an incentive to reassess the suitability of conditions in which your horse is kept, even if others care for your horse in a livery yard. Check for yourself that the food is of good quality and the correct amount is being fed. You will have learned from this book that too much food can be as bad as too little. Everything concerning the well-being of your horse should be looked at, including its exercise regime and the whole environment in which it lives. We have removed the horse from its normal living environment and domesticated it. Therefore we have a responsibility to ensure its lifestyle remains as close to its natural state as possible. Every effort should be made to keep the horse physically and mentally sound. That includes learning everything about the horse's requirements by asking competent experts (not necessarily the farmer next door).

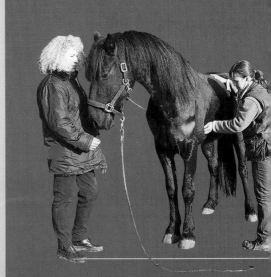